EVERYTHING ABOUT MULTIPLE MYELOMA

A Complete Guide For Patients, Caregivers, And Healthcare Professionals - Causes, Symptoms, Diagnosis, Treatment, Coping Strategies, And More

DR. CADE JOSUE

Table of Contents

DISCLAIMER

The information provided in this book is for general informational purposes only. It is not intended as medical advice, diagnosis, or treatment.

The content of this book should not be considered a substitute for professional medical advice. Readers should consult with a qualified healthcare provider for diagnosis and treatment of any medical conditions they have.

While every effort has been made to ensure the accuracy and completeness of the information presented, the author makes no representations or warranties of any kind, express or implied, about the completeness, accuracy, reliability, suitability, or availability with respect to the information, contained in this book.

The author disclaims any responsibility for any loss or damage resulting from reliance on the information provided in this book. References to individuals, products, websites, organizations, or other names are for informational purposes only and do not imply endorsement.

By reading this book, readers acknowledge that they are responsible for their own health decisions and should seek appropriate medical advice when necessary.

ABOUT THIS BOOK

"Everything About Multiple Myeloma" is an essential reference for researchers, patients, and healthcare professionals, as it offers a thorough comprehension of the intricate and progressively widespread hematologic malignancy known as multiple myeloma.

This book commences with an extensive exposition on multiple myeloma, encompassing its definition, epidemiology, and risk factors; this provision establishes a firm groundwork for the following chapters. By thoroughly examining the pathophysiology, the text clarifies the genetic and molecular foundations of the disease, which are essential for the development of precise therapeutic approaches.

The comprehensive examination of clinical manifestations and symptoms, which are critical for prompt diagnosis, is one of this book's strengths. Distinguishing between advanced imaging studies, laboratory tests, and bone marrow biopsies, the diagnostic approaches section provides readers with the information required to conduct precise evaluations.

Furthermore, the clarification of staging and classification frameworks, such as the Revised International Staging System (R-ISS) and International Staging System (ISS), enables the implementation of standardized approaches to assessing diseases and devising treatments.

A comprehensive discourse regarding treatment modalities highlights the dynamic nature of the therapeutic domain, which includes immunotherapy, stem cell transplantation, chemotherapy, targeted therapies, and targeted therapies.

Constantly emphasized are supportive care and symptom management, which encompass the management of pain, bone health, and nutritional support. By doing so, patients' overall well-being is improved during the course of their illness.

This book effectively addresses complications and prognosis, providing insights into neurological sequelae, infections, and renal complications, in addition to illuminating prognostic factors and survival rates. The text establishes a foundation for improvements in patient care and outcomes through its clarification of forthcoming directions and significant research trends, such as biomarker and novel therapy development.

Moreover, the incorporation of sections addressing coping mechanisms, patient education, and support highlights a comprehensive methodology towards attending to patients, placing equal significance on psychosocial welfare and medicinal interventions.

Fundamentally, "Everything About Multiple Myeloma" functions as an indispensable compilation, furnishing clinicians, researchers, and patients with the requisite information and resources to adeptly navigate the intricacies associated with this hematologic malignancy.

CHAPTER ONE

A Brief Overview Of Multiple Myeloma

Myeloma of multiple varieties is a malignancy that impacts plasma cells, a subset of white blood cells that aids in the immune system's antibody synthesis.

Multiple myeloma is characterized by the uncontrolled multiplication of aberrant plasma cells in the bone marrow, which displaces healthy blood cells. This result in anemia, compromised immune function, and weakened bones, among other complications.

Despite the absence of a remedy for multiple myeloma at present, substantial progress in treatment has resulted in improved prognoses for a considerable number of patients.

Exposition And Synopsis

Myeloma, or multiple myeloma, is an uncommon form of myeloma that affects plasma cells. Plasma cells are an essential component of the immune system, as they generate immunoglobulins (also referred to as antibodies), which aid in the body's defense against infections. In multiple myeloma, myeloma cells, which are aberrant plasma cells, proliferate uncontrollably in the bone marrow, the site of blood cell production.

Myeloma cells have the potential to generate aberrant proteins and develop into malignancies within the bone marrow, thereby instigating a multitude of complications. The proliferation of malignant cells disrupts the synthesis of healthy blood cells, resulting in clinical manifestations including anemia, heightened vulnerability to infections, and complications associated with bone health.

Multiple myeloma is classified as a relatively uncommon malignancy, comprising merely 1% of the total cancer cases and 10% of hematologic malignancies. Multiple myeloma, despite its infrequency, ranks second in terms of prevalence only to non-Hodgkin lymphoma. It predominantly impacts the elderly population, with an average age of diagnosis in the mid-60s.

Aspects Of Epidemiology And Prevalence

Variations in the incidence of multiple myeloma are notable among regions globally, with more developed countries exhibiting comparatively higher rates. An estimated 34,000 new cases of multiple myeloma were identified in the United States in 2020, resulting in approximately 12,000 fatalities attributable to the disease. In contrast, incidence rates have exhibited a gradual ascent in recent decades, plausibly attributable to advancements in detection techniques and the aging of the population.

Additionally, specific demographic variables impact the likelihood of developing multiple myeloma. It occurs more frequently in African Americans than in individuals of other races or ethnicities and is more prevalent in men than in women. Furthermore, age stands as a substantial risk factor, as there is a noticeable rise in the occurrence of multiple myeloma as one grows older.

Factors And Causes Of Risk

Although the precise etiology of multiple myeloma remains unknown, numerous risk factors that may elevate the likelihood of developing the condition have been identified. These consist of:

1. Age: The incidence of multiple myeloma is notably higher among individuals aged 65 and

above, as the disease predominantly affects this demographic.

2. Gender: Multiple myeloma is marginally more prevalent in men than in women.

3. Race: The incidence of multiple myeloma is significantly higher among African Americans in comparison to people of other racial or ethnic backgrounds.

4. Family History: An elevated risk may be associated with having a first-degree relative (e.g., a parent or sibling) diagnosed with multiple myeloma or a related disorder known as monoclonal gammopathy of undetermined significance (MGUS).

5. Prolonged exposure to elevated levels of radiation, such as that which occurs during specific medical procedures or nuclear incidents, has the

potential to elevate the likelihood of developing multiple myeloma.

6. Although the precise mechanism remains unknown, some evidence suggests that obesity may be associated with an increased risk of multiple myeloma.

7. Several studies have proposed a possible correlation between occupational exposure to specific compounds or contaminants and an elevated susceptibility to multiple myeloma. However, further research is required to definitively establish this link.

Mechanisms Underlying Multiple Myeloma

Multiple myeloma is characterized by a complex pathophysiology involving numerous molecular, genetic, and environmental factors.

Multiple myeloma is fundamentally distinguished by an atypical proliferation of plasma cells, resulting in an excessive synthesis of monoclonal immunoglobulins (M proteins) or immunoglobulin fragments.

While the precise chronology of occurrences that culminate in the onset of multiple myeloma remains elusive, speculation suggests that it consists of a succession of genetic mutations that interfere with the typical control of cellular proliferation and viability. Genes that regulate, among other processes, DNA repair, apoptosis (programmed cell death), and cell cycle progression are susceptible to these mutations.

Multiple myeloma is distinguished by the existence of genetic abnormalities, such as deletions, translocations, and mutations of chromosomes.

These irregularities have the potential to disrupt numerous cellular pathways that are implicated in the processes of cell survival, proliferation, and interaction with the microenvironment of the bone marrow.

Multiple myeloma pathogenesis is significantly influenced by the bone marrow microenvironment, which provides a favorable environment for the survival and proliferation of myeloma cells. Myeloma cells engage in interactions with diverse cellular constituents, such as stromal cells, osteoclasts (which are responsible for bone resorption), osteoblasts (which are involved in bone formation), cytokines, and growth factors, within the bone marrow.

These interactions stimulate the production of factors that contribute to bone destruction and the development of other complications associated with multiple myeloma, while also promoting the proliferation of myeloma cells and inhibiting their apoptosis.

In general, the pathogenesis of multiple myeloma involves intricate interactions among dysregulated cellular pathways, genetic abnormalities, and the microenvironment of the bone marrow.

It is imperative to comprehend these mechanisms to advance the creation of targeted therapies that can efficaciously address this arduous ailment.

CHAPTER TWO

Basis In Genetics And Molecular

1. Clonal Expansion: The development of multiple myeloma is initiated by an uncontrolled proliferation of plasma cells within a solitary clone. The process of clonal expansion is propelled by molecular dysregulations and genetic alterations.

2. Chromosomal abnormalities are of considerable importance in the development of multiple myeloma, as they involve genetic factors. Chromosome translocations, deletions, and amplifications are examples.

Chondrosoma 13, 14, and 17, in addition to the immunoglobulin heavy chain (IGH) locus, are frequently implicated in chromosomal abnormalities associated with multiple myeloma.

3. Recurrent translocations involving the IGH locus result in the dysregulation of oncogenes that promote cell survival and proliferation, including MYC, MAF, and CCND1.

4. Tumor suppressor genes, including TP53 and RB1, are implicated in the progression of certain diseases through their deletion or mutation, which facilitates unrestricted cell proliferation and genomic instability.

5. Microenvironmental Interactions: The survival and proliferation of myeloma cells are significantly influenced by the bone marrow microenvironment.

Discourse and therapeutic response are influenced by cytokines and growth factors in the microenvironment, and interactions between myeloma cells and stromal cells.

Advancement And Development

1. MGUS is a condition that serves as a precursor to multiple myeloma. It is distinguished by the presence of a monoclonal protein (M protein) in the bloodstream in the absence of any indications of end-organ injury. Over time, MGUS may transform into either indolent multiple myeloma or multiple myeloma.

2. Smoldering multiple myeloma (SMM) is characterized by elevated concentrations of M protein and plasma cells in comparison to MGUS; however, patients with SMM do not manifest any symptoms or end-organ injury. A greater risk of progression to active multiple myeloma is associated with SMM.

3. Active multiple myeloma is distinguished by the manifestation of clinical symptoms including lytic bone lesions, bone pain, anemia, and renal dysfunction. As the disease advances, the tumor

burden increases, treatment resistance develops, and complications such as infections and renal failure manifest.

4. Relapse and Refractory Disease: Multiple myeloma frequently recurs or develops resistance to therapy despite initial responses to treatment. This can be attributed to factors such as clonal evolution, the emergence of drug resistance, and microenvironment-mediated mechanisms.

Clinical Symptoms And Manifestations

1. Osteomyelitis-Associated Bone Pain: Lytic bone lesions, which result from myeloma cell infiltration into the bone marrow, may induce skeletal complications including fractures and bone pain.

2. Anemia: Plasma cell infiltration into the bone marrow can disrupt regular hematopoiesis, resulting in fatigue and anemia.

3. Renal Dysfunction and Failure: Numerous mechanisms by which the production of monoclonal proteins can induce kidney injury can result in renal dysfunction and failure.

4. Hypercalcemia is a condition characterized by elevated calcium levels in the bloodstream, which are caused by increased bone resorption caused by myeloma cells. Symptoms include weakness, confusion, and constipation.

5. Immunodeficiency: Patients diagnosed with multiple myeloma are at an increased risk of contracting infections, specifically urinary tract infections and bacterial pneumonia.

6. Neurological Symptoms: In rare instances, neurological symptoms such as numbness, lethargy, or paralysis may be induced by myeloma-related amyloidosis or compression of neural structures upon bone lesions.

Diagnostic Methodologies

1. Protein electrophoresis of serum and urine: Identifies the existence of M proteins, which are monoclonal, in the blood or urine. These proteins serve as an indicator of plasma cell dyscrasias, such as multiple myeloma.

2. Bone Marrow Aspiration and Biopsy: The analysis of bone marrow samples enables the detection of cytogenetic abnormalities, infiltration of plasma cells, and determination of the disease burden.

3. Utilizing X-rays, CT scans, MRI scans, and PET scans, imaging studies assess the extent of the disease, monitor the patient's response to treatment, and detect lytic bone lesions.

4. Laboratory tests such as the complete blood count (CBC), serum chemistry, and renal function tests are utilized to evaluate metabolic

abnormalities linked to multiple myeloma, including but not limited to anemia, renal dysfunction, and hypercalcemia.

5. Cytogenetic and molecular testing encompass the utilization of fluorescence in situ hybridization (FISH) and molecular profiling techniques to detect genetic mutations and chromosomal abnormalities that are correlated with treatment response and disease prognosis.

6. International Myeloma Working Group (IMWG) Criteria: The diagnosis and risk stratification of multiple myeloma and its precursor conditions are determined by clinical and laboratory criteria, which include specific biomarkers and the presence of end-organ damage.

It is critical to comprehend the genetic, molecular, and clinical dimensions of multiple myeloma to enhance patient outcomes through precise diagnosis, prognosis evaluation, and individualized therapeutic approaches. Further investigation into the molecular processes that contribute to the advancement of this difficult disease and the emergence of drug resistance continues to provide valuable insights for the creation of innovative targeted therapies and immunotherapies.

CHAPTER THREE

Imaging Research Regarding Multiple Myeloma

Imaging studies are of paramount importance in the identification, progression, and surveillance of multiple myeloma (MM), a hematologic cancer distinguished by the proliferation of atypical plasma cells within the bone marrow. By detecting complications, evaluating bone involvement, and informing treatment decisions, these imaging modalities are of great assistance. The principal imaging modalities employed in the diagnosis of multiple myeloma comprise:

1. X-rays (Radiography): When assessing skeletal involvement in MM, X-rays are frequently the initial imaging modality utilized. Lytic lesions, fractures, and bone degeneration, which are characteristic features of the disease, may become apparent. Nevertheless, the accuracy of X-

ray detection of early bone lesions and assessment of bone marrow involvement may be compromised.

2. Computed tomography (CT) scans are valuable for detecting complications such as fractures or spinal cord compression, evaluating bone lesions, and determining the extent of disease involvement. They produce detailed cross-sectional images of the body. Additionally, CT imaging can aid in the detection of extramedullary disease and the assessment of treatment response.

3. Magnetic Resonance Imaging (MRI): Detecting soft tissue lesions and bone marrow involvement in MM with MRI is a highly sensitive process. It is especially advantageous in the evaluation of spinal cord compression, assessment of bone marrow infiltration, and detection of focal lesions that are not discernible through X-ray or CT imaging. In MM, whole-body MRI has emerged as a

potentially useful instrument for comprehensive disease evaluation.

4. Positron Emission Tomography-Computed Tomography (PET-CT): Active myeloma lesions and other regions of elevated metabolic activity are detected using PET-CT, which combines functional imaging with anatomical data. Its utility extends to the evaluation of treatment response, identification of disease recurrence, and differentiation of benign lesions, including degenerative changes, from active disease.

5. A bone scan, also known as bone scintigraphy, is a diagnostic procedure in which a radioactive tracer is injected and accumulates in regions of heightened bone turnover, such as lytic lesions observed in multiple myeloma. Although bone scans are utilized less frequently than other imaging modalities, they can be utilized to evaluate overall skeletal burden and detect multifocal bone involvement.

6. Although ultrasonography is not commonly utilized in the evaluation of MM, it can be employed to guide procedures like bone marrow biopsy and to assess complications like renal involvement.

To monitor the response to therapy, guide treatment decisions, and comprehensively assess the extent of disease involvement, patients with multiple myeloma frequently undergo a combination of imaging studies.

Biopsy Of Bone Marrow In Multiple Myeloma

A bone marrow biopsy (BMB) is an indispensable diagnostic procedure utilized to assess the presence of multiple myeloma (MM). The procedure entails the removal and analysis of bone marrow tissue to determine the extent of bone marrow involvement, identify the presence of abnormal plasma cells, and assess for additional hematologic abnormalities. The following is a synopsis of the procedure and its importance in MM:

1. Method: A bone marrow biopsy involves a healthcare provider anesthetizing the epidermis and underlying tissue above the hipbone (posterior iliac crest) before extracting a small sample of bone marrow and bone tissue with a specialized instrument. Although mild discomfort may be experienced, the procedure is generally well tolerated.

2. Plasma Cell Evaluation: The bone marrow sample acquired from the biopsy is subjected to microscopic examination to determine the proportion of plasma cells that are present. MM is characterized by an increase in aberrant plasma cells, which have the potential to aggregate or spread in sheets, displacing healthy hematopoietic cells.

3. Evaluation of Bone Marrow Microenvironment: Bone marrow biopsy provides an opportunity to assess the bone marrow microenvironment, encompassing factors such as fibrosis, angiogenesis, and the interplay between plasma cells and supportive stromal cells, in addition to evaluating plasma cell infiltration.

4. Cytogenetic and molecular analyses may be performed on bone marrow biopsy samples to detect genetic alterations such as gene mutations, chromosomal abnormalities, and others that could potentially impact the prognosis of the disease and the response to treatment.

5. Staging and Prognostication: For staging and prognostication in MM, the results of a bone marrow biopsy, including the percentage of plasma cells, cytogenetic abnormalities, and other characteristics, are crucial. They assist in risk group classification for patients and direct treatment decisions.

6. Monitoring Response to Treatment: To evaluate response and disease progression, repeat bone marrow biopsies may be performed throughout the course of treatment. A resolution of bone marrow infiltration or a reduction in the proportion of plasma cells signifies a positive response to the treatment.

In its entirety, bone marrow biopsy serves as a fundamental component in the identification, classification, and control of multiple myeloma, imparting significant insights into the extent of the disease, prognostic elements, and efficacy of treatment.

Systems For Staging And Classification Of Multiple Myeloma

In the field of multiple myeloma (MM), staging and classification systems play a critical role in various aspects, including disease severity stratification, prognosis prediction, and treatment decision guidance for patients. Numerous staging systems have been devised to evaluate diverse facets of MM, encompassing disease biology, clinical manifestations, and tumor burden. The International Staging System (ISS) and the Revised International Staging System (R-ISS) are two staging systems that are extensively utilized. Let us thoroughly examine each of these systems:

1. ISS: International Staging System

• The ISS, which was established in 2005, exclusively relies on two laboratory parameters: albumin and beta-2 microglobulin (β2M) in the serum.

• Patients are categorized into three distinct phases according to the following criteria:

• Serum 2M $\leq$ 3.5 mg/L and serum albumin $\geq$ 3.5 g/dL constitute Stage I.

• Stage II: The criteria for stages I and III were not fulfilled.

• Stage III: Serum 2M concentration greater than or equal to 5.5 mg/L

• Although the ISS offers a straightforward and replicable approach to risk stratification in MM, it is constrained in its ability to capture additional prognostic factors.

2. R-ISS: Revised International Staging System

• The R-ISS, which was introduced in 2015, augments serum 2M and albumin with additional prognostic factors.

In conjunction with the aforementioned parameters, the R-ISS encompasses cytogenetic abnormalities identified via fluorescence in situ hybridization (FISH) and serum lactate dehydrogenase (LDH) levels.

• based on combinations of these factors, patients are categorized into one of three risk categories (R-ISS I, R-ISS II, and R-ISS III), which offers a more precise method of risk stratification in comparison to the ISS.

• By facilitating a more comprehensive evaluation of disease biology and prognosis, the R-ISS contributes to the improvement of treatment planning and patient counseling.

The Durie-Salmon Staging System, which takes tumor burden into account, and the International Myeloma Working Group (IMWG) criteria for designating high-risk disease are additional staging systems utilized in MM.

In patients with multiple myeloma, these staging systems—including the ISS and R-ISS—are indispensable instruments for clinicians to use in risk stratification, treatment selection, and prognosis.

CHAPTER FOUR

System Of Durie-Salmon Staging

The Durie-Salmon Staging System was among the initial staging systems to be specifically designed for the management of multiple myeloma. It assists medical professionals in evaluating the degree of disease advancement and prognosis, thereby facilitating treatment strategizing and patient care. The system assesses three fundamental factors:

1. Tumor Burden: This metric evaluates the number of atypical plasma cells that are present within the organism, taking into account variables such as tumor size, the number of bone lesions, and the existence of supplementary tumors.

2. Monoclonal protein (M protein), which is found in the serum, is an aberrant protein that is generated by myeloma

cells. The quantity of M protein detected in the blood, as assessed by immunofixation electrophoresis (IFE) or serum protein electrophoresis (SPEP), is taken into account by the staging system.

3. Hemoglobin and calcium levels serve as indicators of the extent to which myeloma affects the composition of the blood and the metabolism of calcium. Hypocalcemia, characterized by elevated blood calcium levels, and low hemoglobin levels (anemia) are frequent complications of multiple myeloma and are incorporated into the staging system.

The patients are classified into stages I, II, or III according to these factors; each stage corresponds to a worsening prognosis and a greater severity of the disease.

The information provided by this staging system is of great value in influencing treatment decisions and forecasting patient outcomes.

Therapeutic Modalities

In most cases, multiple myeloma is managed with a combination of therapies that are customized to the particular circumstances of each patient. Treatment selection is contingent upon a variety of elements, including the patient's general well-being, the stage of the disease, genetic predispositions, and treatment objectives. Frequent treatment modalities consist of:

1. Chemotherapy: Chemotherapy is the use of medicines to either eliminate or halt the development of cancer cells. It is frequently a fundamental component of treatment for multiple myeloma and can be administered via oral or intravenous route.

Chemotherapy regimens may comprise proteasome inhibitors, immunomodulatory agents, corticosteroids, alkylating agents, and other drug combinations.

2. Immunotherapy: By utilizing the immune system, immunotherapy targets and destroys cancer cells. Adoptive cell therapies, immune checkpoint inhibitors, and monoclonal antibodies are all examples of immunotherapeutic approaches utilized in the treatment of multiple myeloma. By targeting specific molecules in cancer cells or boosting the activity of immune cells to combat the disease, these treatments are possible.

3. Targeted Therapies: Designed to inhibit the activity of particular molecules or pathways that are essential for the survival and proliferation of malignancy. NF-κB, a critical pathway in the proliferation and survival of myeloma cells, or proteins such as CD38, which are extensively

expressed in myeloma cells, may be the targets of targeted therapies in multiple myeloma.

4.   Stem   cell transplantation, specifically autologous stem cell transplantation (ASCT), represents a viable therapeutic alternative for patients who meet the eligibility criteria and are diagnosed with multiple myeloma. The process consists of harvesting healthy stem cells from the patient, destroying malignant cells with high-dose chemotherapy, and then reinfusing the harvested stem cells to restore blood cell production.

5. Supportive therapies are indispensable in conjunction with anti-myeloma treatments to effectively manage symptoms and complications that may arise during the course of the disease. Antibiotics to prevent infections, pain management, bisphosphonate therapy to prevent bone complications, and blood transfusions to treat anemia are some examples.

The Use Of Chemotherapy

The utilization of chemotherapy is essential in the management of multiple myeloma. It entails the administration of cytotoxic medications to eliminate or impede the development of cancer cells. Multiple myeloma chemotherapy regimens frequently combine medications with distinct mechanisms of action to maximize efficacy and reduce the risk of resistance.

The following chemotherapy medications are frequently employed to treat multiple myeloma:

1. Melphalan is an alkylating agent that induces cell apoptosis by interfering with DNA replication.

2. Bortezomib (Velcade) is a proteasome inhibitor that induces apoptosis (cell death) by interfering with protein degradation in myeloma cells.

3. Lenalidomide (Revlimid) and Pomalidomide (Pomalyst) are immunomodulatory drugs (IMiDs)

that inhibit the proliferation of myeloma cells while enhancing immune function.

4. Dexamethasone, an anti-inflammatory and immunosuppressive corticosteroid, is frequently administered in conjunction with other medications to augment their efficacy.

Oral or intravenous administration of chemotherapy is possible, contingent upon the particular medications and treatment protocol involved. Cycles are commonly employed, wherein treatment intervals are succeeded by periods of leisure to facilitate the body's recuperation from adverse effects.

Chemotherapy has the potential to eradicate cancer cells; however, it also engenders adverse effects including fatigue, hair loss, vertigo, and heightened vulnerability to infections.

The Use Of Immunotherapy

As an effective method for treating multiple myeloma, immunotherapy utilizes the immune system to identify and eliminate malignant cells. Numerous immunotherapeutic approaches have demonstrated effectiveness in the treatment of multiple myeloma:

1. Monoclonal antibodies are molecules manufactured in the laboratory with the ability to selectively bind to proteins that are expressed on the surface of myeloma cells. In the case of daratumumab and elotuzumab, which target the CD38 and SLAMF7 (CS1) proteins, respectively, myeloma cells are destroyed via immune-mediated mechanisms.

2. Immune checkpoint inhibitors function by impeding inhibitory pathways, which are responsible for the suppression of immune cell activity. Although these compounds have

demonstrated efficacy in treating other types of malignancy, their potential in the context of multiple myeloma remains under investigation.

3. CAR T-cell Therapy: To implement CAR T-cell therapy, the T cells of a patient are genetically modified to express chimeric antigen receptors, which are designed to identify particular proteins present in cancer cells. Subsequently, the patient is infused with these modified T cells, which are capable of selectively eliminating myeloma cells. Positive results have been observed in clinical trials evaluating CAR T-cell therapy for multiple myeloma, especially in patients with relapsed or resistant disease.

Immunotherapy presents the capacity to elicit long-lasting responses and mitigate toxicity in contrast to conventional chemotherapy. As with other cancer treatments, however, infusion reactions, cytokine release syndrome, and immune-related adverse events are possible side effects.

Concentrated Therapies

Targeted therapies are specifically formulated to disrupt particular molecules or pathways that are implicated in the progression and viability of multiple myeloma. Targeted therapies have the potential to enhance treatment efficacy and reduce toxicity by selectively eliminating cancer cells while sparing healthy cells by exploiting these particular vulnerabilities. Numerous targeted therapies for multiple myeloma have been devised, including:

1. Proteasome inhibitors, including bortezomib, carfilzomib, and ixazomib, selectively interact with the proteasome, an intracellular complex that is tasked with the degradation of proteins. Adopting an apoptosis-inducing mechanism, these pharmaceuticals disrupt protein

homeostasis within myeloma cells by inhibiting proteasome activity.

2. Immunomodulatory Drugs (IMiDs): IMiDs, such as lenalidomide and pomalidomide, inhibit the proliferation and survival of myeloma cells and modulate the immune system. They also possess antiangiogenic properties.

3. Monoclonal antibodies, including daratumumab and elotuzumab, selectively bind to proteins that are expressed on the myeloma cell surface. This results in the eradication of malignancy cells via immune-mediated mechanisms.

4. Histone deacetylase (HDAC) inhibitors, including belinostat, panobinostat, and vorinostat, exert their effects by selectively targeting enzymes implicated in epigenetic regulation. Consequently, these inhibitors perturb gene expression, which in

turn impedes the proliferation of myeloma cells and triggers apoptosis.

5. BCL-2 Inhibitors: Proteins implicated in the regulation of apoptosis are targeted by BCL-2 inhibitors, including venetoclax, which induces programmed cell death in myeloma cells.

Combining targeted therapies with additional anti-myeloma agents, such as immunotherapy or chemotherapy, is also possible. These treatments present the possibility of enhanced accuracy and efficacy, especially for individuals who have specific genetic abnormalities or have developed resistance to traditional therapies.

As a result of its heterogeneity and complexity, multiple myeloma necessitates a multidisciplinary treatment approach. Treatment decisions are guided by staging systems such as the Durie-Salmon Staging System, which aids clinicians in determining the severity of a disease. A variety of treatment modalities are available to address multiple myeloma, comprising immunotherapy, targeted therapies, chemotherapy, and immunotherapy. Each of these approaches has distinct mechanisms of action and potential advantages. Healthcare providers can optimize patient outcomes for multiple myeloma by comprehending and incorporating these concepts into their clinical practice.

CHAPTER FIVE

Cell Stem Transplantation

Multiple myeloma is frequently treated with bone marrow transplantation, also referred to as stem cell transplantation. A healthy blood-forming stem cell infusion is utilized to replace diseased or damaged bone marrow within the body. In the treatment of multiple myeloma, two primary varieties of stem cell transplantation are utilized:

1. Autologous stem cell transplantation involves the collection of stem cells from the patient's blood or bone marrow before the commencement of treatment.

Following the administration of high-dose chemotherapy to eradicate malignant cells, the gathered stem cells are reintroduced into the patient's circulatory system to facilitate the regeneration of robust bone marrow.

2. Allogeneic stem cell transplantation involves the procurement of stem cells from a donor whose tissue type is highly compatible with that of the recipient. A greater risk of complications, including graft-versus-host disease (GVHD), in which the donor cells invade the recipient's tissues, is associated with allogeneic transplants.

The goal of stem cell transplantation is to restore the bone marrow's capacity to generate healthy blood cells by eradicating malignant cells. It has the potential to increase survival rates and prolong remission periods, especially in younger patients and those afflicted with aggressive forms of the disease.

Supportive Care And Management Of Symptoms

Improving the quality of life and managing multiple myeloma patients requires the provision of essential supportive care. A multidisciplinary approach is incorporated to examine the disease's impacts on physical, emotional, and social well-being, among other facets. The following are essential elements of supportive care:

• Routine Monitoring: Thorough surveillance of the advancement of the disease via diagnostic imaging modalities, blood tests, and bone marrow biopsies enables prompt modifications to be made to treatment strategies.

• Pain Management: Bone pain may be induced by multiple myeloma as a result of bone lesions and fractures. In addition to radiation therapy and nerve blocks, pain management strategies may involve the use of nonsteroidal anti-inflammatory medicines (NSAIDs), analgesics, and bisphosphonates.

• Administration of Anemia and Fatigue: Anemia, which results in frailty and fatigue, is a prevalent complication of multiple myeloma. Blood transfusions or erythropoiesis-stimulating agents (ESAs) to replenish hemoglobin levels may be utilized in the course of treatment to induce red blood cell production.

• Infection Prevention and Treatment: The immune system of patients with multiple myeloma and its treatments may be compromised, rendering them more vulnerable to infections. Antimicrobial prophylaxis, vaccinations, and prompt treatment of infections are critical.

• Psychosocial Support: The emotional and mental toll of coping with a cancer diagnosis can be significant. Patients and their families can benefit from psychosocial support, which consists of educational materials, counseling, and support groups, to assist them in coping with the emotional effects of the disease and its treatment.

Anxiety Management

As bone pain is a prevalent symptom of multiple myeloma, pain management is an essential component of patient care. Pain management aims to increase function, alleviate discomfort, and enhance quality of life.

Analgesic medications are frequently prescribed to patients with multiple myeloma to alleviate discomfort. Nonsteroidal anti-inflammatory drugs (NSAIDs), analgesics, and adjuvant medications (e.g., anticonvulsants or depressants) for neuropathic pain are examples of such substances.

• Bisphosphonates: Bisphosphonates, a class of medications, assist in the prevention of fractures and the reinforcement of bones in multiple myeloma patients. Additionally, they can mitigate bone discomfort through the inhibition of osteoclast activity, which is a cell responsible for the degradation of bone tissue.

• Radiation Therapy: To target specific areas of bone pain caused by multiple myeloma, radiation therapy may be utilized. It aids in the reduction of pain, alleviates pressure on nerves, and shrinks tumors.

Nerve blocks are a potential treatment option for severe pain that has not shown improvement with alternative methods. They function by momentarily impeding the transmission of pain signals to the brain. In this procedure, anesthetic or anti-inflammatory drugs are injected near the neurons that are accountable for pain transmission.

• Physical Therapy: Strength, flexibility, and mobility can be enhanced through exercise and physical therapy, thereby alleviating pain and improving overall health. Personalized exercise regimens that account for an individual's unique capabilities and constraints may additionally aid in fatigue management and mood enhancement.

Bone Wellness

Patients with multiple myeloma must prioritize bone health maintenance due to the disease's propensity to compromise bone integrity and elevate the likelihood of fractures. The following are strategies for promoting bone health:

• Bisphosphonates: Patients diagnosed with multiple myeloma frequently undergo treatment with bisphosphonate medications, including zoledronic acid and pamidronate, to mitigate the risk of fractures and prevent bone loss. By inhibiting the activity of osteoclasts, which degrade bone tissue, these drugs are effective.

• Supplementation with Calcium and Vitamin D: Sufficient consumption of calcium and vitamin D is critical for the preservation of bone density and strength. Supplementation may be necessary for patients diagnosed with multiple myeloma, particularly those undergoing treatment involving bisphosphonates that have the potential to disrupt calcium metabolism.

Weight-bearing exercises regularly, including jogging, walking, and resistance training, can aid in bone strengthening and fracture prevention. In addition to enhancing general health and well-being, physical activity aids in the preservation of muscular strength and equilibrium.

• Fall Prevention: Patients with compromised bone strength are particularly susceptible to falls, which present a substantial hazard.

Removing trip hazards from the home environment, utilizing assistive devices such as hold bars and handrails, and engaging in balance exercises are all preventative measures against falls.

• Cessation of Smoking and Alcohol Limitation: Excessive alcohol consumption and smoking can have detrimental effects on bone health. By quitting smoking and limiting alcohol consumption, the risk of fractures can be reduced and bones can be better protected.

CHAPTER SIX

Nutritional Assistance

The administration of nutritional support is crucial in the management of multiple myeloma and in promoting general health and well-being. Nutritional deficiencies may manifest in patients diagnosed with multiple myeloma as a result of various factors, including reduced appetite, treatment-related adverse effects, and malabsorption. Methods of providing nutritional support consist of:

A balanced diet comprises a variety of nutritious components, including fruits, vegetables, whole cereals, lean proteins, and healthy lipids. This composition is crucial for sustaining energy, promoting overall health, and facilitating immune function. Additionally, proper hydration is essential for sustaining kidney function and preventing dehydration.

• Supplementation: Nutritional supplements may be advised in certain instances to rectify particular deficiencies. Patients suffering from anemia, for instance, might benefit from iron supplements, whereas those suffering from vitamin D deficiency might necessitate vitamin D supplementation.

• Nutrition Counseling: By seeking guidance from a registered dietitian, patients can optimize their dietary regimen to address treatment-related adverse effects, including vertigo, vomiting, and changes in flavor, while also ensuring that their nutritional requirements are met.

• Monitoring and Assessment: Consistent monitoring of nutritional status, encompassing body composition, weight, and laboratory indicators of nutritional status, can facilitate the timely detection of insufficiencies and inform preventive interventions against potential complications.

• Supportive Care: Antiemetic medications for the management of nausea and vomiting, appetite stimulants, and dietary modifications are examples of supportive care measures that can assist patients with multiple myeloma in enhancing their nutritional intake and quality of life.

Consequences And Prognosis

Complicated Bones:

Multiple myeloma frequently manifests as bone discomfort, a condition that can significantly impair an individual's mobility and overall quality of life.

• Bone Fractures: Even with minimal trauma, the compromised bones caused by myeloma cell infiltration are susceptible to fractures.

• Hypercalcemia: Disruption of bone tissue can result in elevated blood calcium levels, which can give rise to various symptoms including fatigue, bewilderment, and renal complications.

Anemia (H 0):

Anemia, which is characterized by a reduction in red blood cells, may result in chronic fatigue and frailty.

Adverse Renal Reactions:

• Renal Failure: Patients diagnosed with multiple myeloma frequently experience renal complications as a result of the cancer cells' production of aberrant proteins (light chains), which accumulate and cause kidney injury and potentially renal failure.

• Hypercalcemia-Related Nephropathy: Renal complications can be further aggravated by direct harm to the kidneys caused by elevated calcium levels.

Renal tubular acidosis is a condition that arises when myeloma hinders the kidney's capacity to regulate acid-base equilibrium, thereby causing metabolic acidosis.

Pathogens: Infections

• Immunosuppression: The immune system is compromised as a result of multiple myeloma, which elevates the susceptibility to infections, specifically bacterial pneumonia, urinary tract infections, and sepsis.

• Reactivation of Viral Infections: Due to their compromised immune systems, patients diagnosed with multiple myeloma are more susceptible to viral infections, including herpes zoster (shingles) and cytomegalovirus (CMV).

• Pneumocystis jirovecii Pneumonia (PCP): Individuals undergoing immunosuppressive therapy are susceptible to opportunistic infections such as PCP, a fungal-induced severe lung infection.

Neurological Disorders

• Peripheral neuropathy: Certain patients may experience paralysis, numbness, or sensation in the extremities as a result of peripheral neuropathy; this condition may be caused by nerve injury induced by the disease or specific treatments such as chemotherapy.

Spinal cord compression can result from bone lesions associated with myeloma, which may cause neurological impairments including weakness, numbness, or paralysis in the regions affected.

Hypercalcemia-Associated Neurological Symptoms: Symptoms such as perplexity, lethargy, and coma may result from the impact of elevated calcium levels on the neurological system.

Early Prognosis:

The prognosis for multiple myeloma is highly variable and is influenced by age, genetic abnormalities of the cancer cells, the stage at which the disease is detected, and the overall health of the patient. Recent developments in treatment, such as novel immunotherapies and targeted therapies, have improved the prognosis for a great number of patients. Multiple myeloma continues to be intractable, with variable long-term survival rates. The Revised International Staging System (R-ISS) and International Staging System (ISS) are frequently employed in treatment decision-making and prognosis evaluation.

Aspects That Impact The Prognosis:

The prognosis for patients diagnosed with advanced stages of multiple myeloma is typically less favorable.

Cytogenetic abnormalities, including translocations involving the immunoglobulin heavy chain gene (IGH) or deletion of chromosome 17 (del17p), have been linked to an increased likelihood of disease progression and unfavorable outcomes.

• Treatment Response: Long-term prognoses are generally more favorable for patients who attain a complete or very excellent partial response to initial therapy.

• Age and General Health: Prognoses are generally more favorable for younger patients and those with a reduced number of comorbidities.

Strategies For Treatment:

• Induction therapy is the primary approach utilized to attain remission and decrease tumor burden. It commonly incorporates a combination of immunomodulatory medications (IMiDs), proteasome inhibitors, chemotherapy, and steroids.

• Stem Cell Transplantation: To further solidify response and enhance outcomes, eligible patients may be considered for autologous stem cell transplantation.

• Maintenance therapy may involve the administration of medications such as lenalidomide or bortezomib to certain patients to extend remission and impede the progression of the disease.

• Innovative Therapeutic Agents: Monoclonal antibodies (e.g., elotuzumab and daratumumab), targeted therapies (e.g., ixazomib and carfilzomib), and immunotherapies (e.g., chimeric antigen receptor T-cell therapy) are recent developments in treatment that have expanded patients' treatment options and improved patient outcomes.

Multiple myeloma is, in brief, a multifaceted ailment characterized by a wide array of complications that may impact organ systems such as the nervous system, kidneys, bones, and immune system. Despite recent treatment advancements, the prognosis for patients with multiple myeloma continues to be affected by disease stage, genetic risk factors, and therapeutic response. Strict monitoring and personalized treatment strategies are critical to maximize results and efficiently handle complications.

CHAPTER SEVEN

Factors Prognosticating Multiple Myeloma

Prognostic factors in multiple myeloma are variables that aid in forecasting the probable progression of the illness, encompassing treatment response and overall survival. It is imperative to identify these factors to customize treatment approaches and enhance patient results. A multitude of prognostic factors have been discerned about multiple myeloma; these factors comprise diverse facets of the ailment, such as genetic, laboratory, and clinical attributes.

1. Cytogenetic abnormalities, including but not limited to del(17p), t(4;14), t(14;16), and 1q amplification, are correlated with an unfavorable prognosis in patients with multiple myeloma. Cytogenetic testing is employed to identify these abnormalities, which have a

substantial impact on the process of risk stratification.

2. Serum biomarkers, including lactate dehydrogenase (LDH) and beta-2 microglobulin (β2M), are frequently employed as prognostic indicators due to their quantitative nature. Higher concentrations of these biomarkers are frequently associated with disease progression and unfavorable results.

3. Gene Expression Profiling (GEP): To identify high-risk patients, gene expression profiling techniques analyze patterns of gene activity in myeloma cells. Beyond conventional cytogenetics, GEP assays, such as the 70-gene signature and the UAMS (University of Arkansas for Medical Sciences) classifier, provide vital prognostic information.

4. The International St staging system (ISS) is a widely utilized prognostic instrument that

classifies patients into three distinct risk categories according to their albumin and beta-2 microglobulin serum levels. Patients who are in higher stages of the ISS have a reduced overall survival rate and may necessitate more intensive treatment strategies.

5. Extramedullary disease, characterized by the infiltration of myeloma cells into tissues external to the bone marrow, is correlated with unfavorable results. It frequently signifies a more aggressive course of the disease and resistance to conventional treatments.

6. Age and performance status are patient-related variables that exert an influence on the prognosis. Patients who are elderly or have a low-performance status may exhibit decreased tolerance to intensive treatments, leading to unfavorable outcomes as a result.

7. The evaluation of response to initial therapy, which includes indicators such as the extent and longevity of the response, offers significant prognostic insights. Patients who attain profound and long-lasting responses (e.g., a complete response or an exceptionally favorable partial response) exhibit superior long-term results.

8. Minimal Residual Disease (MRD) is a term used to describe the negligible quantity of cancer cells that persist within the body after treatment, evading traditional detection techniques. A deeper level of response is indicated by MRD negativity, which is associated with increased progression-free and overall survival.

9. Osteolytic lesions and fractures, as well as the extent and severity of bone disease, are significant prognostic indicators in multiple myeloma. A correlation between bone involvement and the aggressiveness of a disease can influence treatment decisions and outcomes.

10. Renal Function: In multiple myeloma, impaired renal function at the time of diagnosis is a negative prognostic factor.

In addition to causing treatment complications, it signifies disease progression and is correlated with decreased survival time.

By recognizing and incorporating these prognostic indicators into clinical practice, risk-adapted treatment approaches can be developed for specific patients, leading to improved outcomes in the context of multiple myeloma.

Ratios Of Survival In Multiple Myeloma

In recent decades, there has been a substantial enhancement in survival rates for individuals with multiple myeloma due to developments in treatment strategies, supportive care, and our comprehension of the disease's biology.

Survival rates for patients diagnosed with multiple myeloma are commonly presented in relative survival, five-year survival, and median survival. These metrics offer valuable insights into the overall prognosis and long-term consequences of the disease.

1. Median Survival: As a result of therapeutic advancements, the median survival for patients diagnosed with multiple myeloma has increased consistently. Historically, the median survival rate was estimated to be between 3 and 4 years. However, that has changed as a result of the development of immunomodulatory drugs and proteasome inhibitors (bortezomib, carfilzomib) and lenalidomide, pomalidomide. Together, these agents have increased median survival to approximately 6-7 years, and in some cases, even longer.

2. The five-year survival rate quantifies the proportion of patients who have maintained their

lives for a period of five years after receiving their diagnosis. At present, the five-year survival rate for newly diagnosed patients with multiple myeloma is approximately 50% to 60%, reflecting a consistent upward trend. Nevertheless, survival rates fluctuate by variables including age, disease stage, and treatment response.

3. Relative Survival: The survival of patients diagnosed with multiple myeloma is compared to that of the general population in terms of relative survival. Age, gender, and the calendar year are some of the variables considered when estimating the excess mortality caused by the disease. The influence of multiple myeloma on survival can be more precisely evaluated using relative survival rates as opposed to overall survival rates.

4. Risk stratification refers to the substantial variation in survival rates that can be attributed to various factors, including patient characteristics, disease stage, and cytogenetic abnormalities.

Clinicians can identify patients with a greater propensity for disease progression and adapt treatment strategies accordingly through the use of risk stratification.

To improve outcomes, high-risk patients might necessitate more intensive therapies or enrollment in clinical trials.

5. The implementation of innovative therapeutic approaches, such as targeted agents, monoclonal antibodies, proteasome inhibitors, and immunomodulatory medications, has been instrumental in elevating the survival rates of individuals afflicted with multiple myeloma. As a result of the increased response rates, protracted remissions, and expanded treatment options brought about by these agents, overall survival rates have improved.

6. The utilization of autologous stem cell transplantation (ASCT) in conjunction with high-

dose chemotherapy continues to be a significant therapeutic approach for patients who meet the eligibility criteria and have multiple myeloma.

In many instances, prolonged survival can result from ASCT-induced profound and long-lasting responses, particularly when combined with novel agents as part of consolidation or upfront therapy.

7. Long-term survivorship is becoming an increasingly prevalent outcome for patients diagnosed with multiple myeloma due to developments in treatment modalities and supportive care.

Long-term survivors encounter distinct obstacles in disease monitoring, treatment-related adverse effects, and quality of life. These challenges underscore the criticality of survivorship care plans and the integration of interdisciplinary assistance.

In general, the prognosis for survival in cases of multiple myeloma has considerably advanced, owing to the influence of developing therapeutic approaches and the increasing focus on personalized medicine methodologies customized to the specific requirements of each patient.

CHAPTER EIGHT

Numerous myelomas

A form of malignancy known as multiple myeloma impacts plasma cells, which are a specific subset of white blood cells responsible for generating antibodies to combat infections.

Multiple myeloma is characterized by the accumulation of aberrant plasma cells in the bone marrow, which displace healthy blood cells and generate atypical proteins. This can result in anemia, compromised immune function, bone injury, and bone deterioration. Although there is currently no cure for multiple myeloma, substantial progress in treatment has led to improved patient outcomes, with many able to effectively manage the condition for years with the appropriate therapies.

Trials In Clinicals

Clinical trials are scientific investigations that assess the efficacy and safety of novel pharmaceuticals, medical treatments, or procedures. Clinical trials are of great significance in the realm of multiple myeloma as they contribute significantly to the advancement of knowledge regarding the disease and the formulation of novel therapeutic approaches. These clinical trials may evaluate novel pharmaceuticals, drug combinations, or alternative treatment modalities, including stem cell transplantation.

Multiple Phases Comprise Clinical Trials

1. Phase I clinical trials are the initial iteration of human testing, during which the safety, dosage, and adverse effects of a novel treatment are determined.

2. Phase II trials assess the treatment's efficacy and safety in a greater number of patients to determine its overall effectiveness.

3. In phase three, comparative trials are conducted to assess the efficacy of the new treatment over the standard treatment. They are essential for determining whether a novel treatment should be approved for extensive use and involve larger patient populations.

4. Phase IV trials are conducted after the treatment's approval and aim to conduct a more comprehensive assessment of its efficacy and safety over an extended period in real-world environments.

Patients who participate in clinical trials may gain access to innovative remedies that would otherwise be unavailable. Nonetheless, it is critical to consider the potential benefits and drawbacks and consult a healthcare professional before proceeding.

Patient Support And Education

Education and support for the patient are essential elements in the management of multiple myeloma. Gaining knowledge regarding the disease, available treatment alternatives, and possible adverse effects provides patients with the agency to make well-informed choices regarding their healthcare and engage actively in the development of their treatment regimen.

Instruction may encompass details about the biological underpinnings of multiple myeloma, treatment options, methods for mitigating symptoms and adverse effects, as well as recommendations for preserving holistic health and wellness.

Support services offer patients and their families emotional, practical, and social assistance during the course of their cancer treatment. Financial assistance, support groups, individual counseling, educational seminars, and assistance traversing the healthcare system are all examples of such services. Support services are designed to assist patients in coping with the physical, emotional, and practical difficulties that may arise as a result of the disease.

Coping Mechanisms

Managing a multiple myeloma diagnosis can present considerable physical and emotional strain. The implementation of efficacious coping mechanisms can assist individuals in controlling tension, diminishing anxiety, and enhancing their holistic well-being. The following may be examples of coping mechanisms utilized by patients with multiple myeloma:

1. Maintaining Knowledge: Acquiring a comprehensive understanding of the ailment, available treatment alternatives and self-care methodologies can assist individuals in feeling more empowered and in charge.

2. Establishing a Support Network: Cultivating a network of empathetic acquaintances, relatives, and medical practitioners can furnish both psychological solace and pragmatic aid.

3. Achieving and Sustaining a Healthy Lifestyle: Tobacco abstinence, excessive alcohol consumption, regular exercise (as prescribed by a healthcare professional), and rest sufficient durations are all components of a healthy lifestyle that contribute to an individual's general health and well-being.

4. Active Engagement in Pleasurable and Relaxing Activities, Enrollment in a Support Group, or Consultation with a Therapist: These pursuits can

assist individuals afflicted with cancer in managing the emotional difficulties that accompany the disease.

5. Establishing Practical Objectives: By concentrating on what is manageable and establishing realistic objectives, one can alleviate feelings of being overwhelmed and sustain a sense of direction and drive.

6. Engaging in Mindfulness and Relaxation Techniques: To alleviate tension and foster relaxation, practitioners may consider incorporating practices such as guided imagery, meditation, yoga, and deep breathing.

7. Participating in Meaningful Activities: Delving into pastimes, passions, and undertakings that elicit delight and satisfaction can offer solace and diversion from the difficulties associated with residing with cancer.

In the end, managing multiple myeloma is a profoundly personal experience, in which strategies that prove effective for one individual may not resonate with another. Patients should investigate and determine which coping mechanisms work best for them, in addition to obtaining support from loved ones and healthcare professionals when necessary.

Summary

In conclusion, patients, caregivers, and healthcare professionals must have a comprehensive understanding of multiple myeloma. This intricate ailment, distinguished by atypical plasma cells within the bone marrow, manifests with an assortment of symptoms and complications that necessitate meticulous attention and therapy. A multidisciplinary approach encompassing oncologists, hematologists, nurses, and supportive care teams is imperative from the moment of initial diagnosis until the provision of ongoing care to maximize patient outcomes and quality of life.

Significant advancements in medical technology and research have transformed the landscape of multiple myeloma treatment. Increasingly inventive targeted therapies and immunotherapies have joined conventional chemotherapy to provide patients with an unprecedented array of treatment options. There is a growing trend toward personalized treatment plans that are customized to the specific disease characteristics and overall health status of each individual. This development provides optimism regarding improved outcomes and extended survival times.

Nevertheless, persistent obstacles persist, encompassing the emergence of drug resistance, the management of treatment-associated adverse effects, and the resolution of the psychosocial ramifications associated with a chronic cancer prognosis. Sustained research endeavors centered on elucidating the fundamental biological mechanisms of multiple myeloma, discovering novel therapeutic targets, and refining supportive care interventions are imperative for the continued improvement of patient outcomes and quality of life.

In summary, although multiple myeloma presents considerable obstacles, continuous progress in both research and clinical application provides optimism regarding forthcoming therapeutic developments and enhanced patient prognoses.

THE END